HEALING WORDS
THE POWER OF APOLOGY IN MEDICINE

MICHAEL S. WOODS, M.D.

HILDA J. BRUCKER
CONTRIBUTING AUTHOR AND RESEARCHER

DOCTORS IN TOUCH
1100 Lake Street, Suite 230
Oak Park, IL 60301

ISBN 0-9755196-0-3

To Marcia,
who has always supported my crazy ideas… and me.

acknowledgements

This book wouldn't exist if not for some very important people and their support, both emotionally and financially. Jim Cunningham is a unique individual who sees the value of and believes in my efforts to enhance the healthcare experience for all stakeholders. There have been many days when, without Jim, I would not have had the energy to continue. His involvement and guidance has suffused me—as well as others—with renewed commitment to our vision. Hilda Brucker, editor, researcher and teacher, has the patience of Job. I contributed the ideas for this work. Hilda went the extra mile—research, telephone calls, e-mails—all to bolster the original ideas. And then she converted what I gave her into the King's English! What I have learned about writing from Hilda cannot be put into words or valued in dollars. Robert Viola and Louis Weisberg, both of communications firm MVTEN, took what I thought was perfect work and made it "perfecter." Louis worked magic with what he calls "tweaks" that added additional clarity and focus without loss of meaning—and, in fact, perhaps added more meaning. Sarah Dore, a fount of reason and a pragmatist who believes in our mission (and apology!), continually challenges me to think differently. Her grasp of the medical malpractice insurance industry is unparalleled. Her sense of humor is nearly as precious as her advice. And my family who, while listed last, are always first. Marcia, my wife, who supported the family while I chased my dream to make a difference. Who never complained about the need for more investment, whether it was my time, or our money. And the one I still love to be with. Our 2-year-old son (who laughs easily and is endlessly curious) and our 1-month-old daughter, remind us daily that there is more to life than money and things. I could live in a refrigerator box with them, as long as I could keep them warm when it was cold, cool when it was hot, and make sure they were never hungry.

In addition to those noted above, others who played a role in this work, in some capacity, include: Sue Ann Capizzi; Lisa Chambers Howard; William Gallagher and Dieter Zimmer of Northwest Physician Mutual in Salem, Ore.; and Ray Mazzotta, Darrell Ranum, and Paul Nagle of OHIC in Columbus, Ohio.

about the author

Dr. Michael S. Woods followed his father's footsteps into medicine, earning an M.D. from the University of Kansas. He completed residency training in general surgery at KU, followed by a fellowship in hepatobiliary-pancreatic surgery at Virginia Mason Clinic in Seattle, Washington.

As a surgeon at the Wichita Clinic in Kansas, Mike became increasingly frustrated by the focus on financial concerns, market competition, and liability issues that were coming to dominate medicine. This was incongruous with the image of healthcare he'd grown up with—the group practice operated by his father and two partners. Their interest was solely in serving their patients. Avoiding malpractice claims was never a concern for them.

Mike went to work for Johnson & Johnson, where within three years he was named Global Medical Leader for clinical research projects supporting one of the largest pharmaceutical programs in the company's history. At Johnson & Johnson, Mike was exposed to personal leadership development, and he was impressed by the success it had in improving customer service and employee satisfaction. Mike immersed himself in the study of this field, which was transforming corporate America. Eventually, he realized that he'd found a concept that could salvage the future of the healthcare system by bringing it back to its roots.

Mike left the pharmaceutical industry in 2001 to write the book "The DEPO Principle: Applying Personal Leadership Principles to Health Care." He also launched a company whose mission is to provide leadership development resources tailored specifically to the needs of doctors, healthcare organizations, and the malpractice insurance industry.

In addition to his consulting work, Mike remains board-certified in surgery and is a fellow of the American College of Surgeons. He is a practicing partner with a surgical group in Colorado, where he resides with his wife Marcia, their son and their newborn daughter, who joined the Woods family on April 1, 2004.

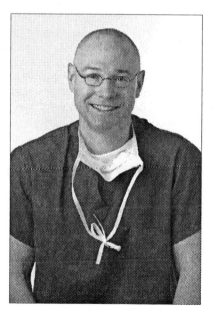

MICHAEL S. WOODS, M.D.

Disclaimer

This material is informational only. Advice given is general. The author does not determine or assume responsibility for how or if an individual chooses to use or not use information contained herein. Physicians should be familiar with their own State laws regarding apology and disclosure, as well as the details of their liability insurance policy regarding apology and/or disclosure. They should contact their liability insurers if they have questions concerning the role of apology and/or disclosure in any situation, prior to speaking with any patient regard an adverse outcome, complication or error. Readers should consult professional counsel for specific legal, ethical, or clinical questions.

table of contents

VIII

introduction

For every medical intervention there is an expected outcome. But there is also the possibility for unintended consequences. While it's comforting to believe modern medical science can perform miracles, the reality is that human bodies often react in unpredictable ways—even when the treatment is standardized and evidence-based.

In this book, I propose that when complications occur, physicians should apologize, offer ongoing care and support, and fully disclose all details to the patient. They should never breach the patient's trust and engage in the kind of cover-ups that have become all too common in healthcare today. This sort of unethical behavior demeans the practice of medicine and fosters a mindset that interferes with our ability to act effectively as healers.

I believe—and statistics support this—that, when dealt with honestly, respectfully, and compassionately, patients will accept an apology and choose not to litigate. Instead, they will accept a fair financial remedy that covers the costs of additional care made necessary by the complication.

What I'm proposing in this book is simple, but profoundly important. I'm encouraging my fellow physicians to practice a common courtesy played out on the street every day.

Just as a stranger automatically apologizes for unintentionally bumping into someone on a sidewalk, an apology should be the norm if a doctor is running late, interrupts a patient to take a phone call, misplaces a file—or initiates care that results in an unexpected or life-threatening outcome.

I believe most physicians long to do the right thing. When one of our patients is in pain, suffers an unanticipated outcome, or fails to respond to treatment, our hearts tell us to empathize, to reach out. Unfortunately, our profession has become increasingly deaf to the calls of the heart. Only we can change this situation.

A word of caution is in order. I believe that saying *I'm sorry* is the right thing to do, and this book contains accurate information on the value of apology in doctor-patient relationships as well as its ability to reduce malpractice claims. Despite this, some malpractice policies are written in such a way that physicians risk loss of coverage by offering an apology or information to a patient without getting prior clearance from the insurer. You must understand what your policy states concerning this issue before following my advice.

Finally, if this book fails to meet the expectations of the reader, I would like to say *I'm sorry* in advance.

reclaiming good medicine

I'm sorry is one of the most commonly used phrases in any language. Few others are applicable to such a wide range of situations. The simple apology is, in fact, something of a rhetorical catchall. It's spoken as a simple act of courtesy when reaching across another person for salt at the dinner table. It's presented as a plea to judges before sentencing is pronounced. It's offered as an expression of sympathy to the bereaved.

For most people, *I'm sorry* is spoken almost reflexively throughout the day to express respect, regret, compassion. Depending on the situation and the way it's said, an apology can be everything from a throwaway social nicety to a profound utterance from the heart.

Yet for us physicians, the words *I'm sorry* are among the hardest to pronounce. In our professional situation, they are fraught with serous ramifications and nuances that other people never have to consider. In many ways, they are words that separate us from the rest of the human race.

During our training, we are taught that we must be infallible—that we cannot make mistakes. Our educations drill into us that data are absolute, that facts allow us to explain outcomes in a linear fashion and figure odds with some measure of precision. But no matter how much comfort we take in the scientific method, the simple truth remains that life is DUN: dynamic, unpredictable, and non-linear. Chaos theory demonstrates that the possibility always exists for unintended consequences. Thus, our schooling sets us up to deny the failure that is embedded in our discipline.

> The simple truth remains that life is DUN: dynamic, unpredictable, and non-linear. Thus, our schooling sets us up to deny the failure that is embedded in our discipline.

As practitioners, insurers tell us that an apology might be interpreted as an admission of fault or negligence that could expose us to litigation. Some insurers will even void the policy of a doctor who apologizes to a patient in the wake of a complication or error.

So it's not surprising that the culture of medicine has evolved to be apology-avoidant. I propose that the health-care profession should take a fresh look at apology—why it is important, how to recognize when it is needed, and how it should be delivered. All of this must be examined within the context of "authentic apology"—that is, apology that is heart-felt and offered because it is the right thing to do—and not apology as a technique to manipulate and placate an angry patient to avoid a lawsuit.

As healers we must also recognize that apology is good medicine that has restorative powers. We must reclaim our right to say *I'm sorry*, because we owe it to our patients. They have a fundamental human need to hear an apology when something goes awry, whether it was directly caused by us or not. In the wake of a bad outcome, saying *I'm sorry* could be as helpful for the patient's—and the physician's—psychic healing process as antibiotics are for curing an infection. This simple but eloquent phrase of compassion is as essential to a doctor's medicine bag as the stethoscope and tongue depressor.

Ironically, despite the warnings of some insurers, data indicate that the likelihood of a lawsuit falls by 50 percent when an apology is offered and the details of a medical error are disclosed immediately. Considering our profession's urgent need to protect itself from medical malpractice liability and considering the near-anarchy over tort reform to limit jury awards, you'd think doctors would be eager to adopt a risk management strategy that offers a 50-percent reduction in litigation.

But unfortunately medicine's difficulty with apology is symptomatic of a much larger communication crisis in healthcare. The environment in which doctors operate today—both literally and figuratively—makes it difficult for us to maintain our focus on the very reason we entered the field in the first place: to serve humanity. We begin learning detachment from the moment we begin medical school, and that attitude is reinforced by a system that demands practicing physicians to see more patients in less time and to be wary of engaging with them in honest, open dialogue.

3

That's unfortunate, because the quality of our communication with patients affects every aspect of the care we provide. And it has a direct bearing on our job satisfaction as well.

Why Patients Really Sue Their Doctors

In 1993, Wendy Levinson, M.D., and her colleagues designed a research study they hoped would show a link between physician-patient communication and the risk of malpractice. They analyzed audiotapes of routine office visits with two groups of physicians: those who had never been sued and those with two or more malpractice suits filed against them.

Levinson found that the physicians with the best communication skills were also those who had not been sued. The former tended to ask more questions, encourage patients to talk about their feelings, use humor when appropriate, and educate patients about what to expect during treatment. These physicians also spent more time per visit with patients than those who had been sued. In fact, the length of office visits alone was strongly correlated with a physician's history of malpractice claims. How much extra time, on average, did the doctors who had never been sued spend with their patients? Three minutes.

Another group of physician researchers studied transcripts of legal depositions given by patients who had filed lawsuits. All of the transcripts included the question *Why are you suing the doctor?* The study concluded that 71 percent of the patient-plaintiffs had had problematic relationships with their physicians before the incidents prompting the lawsuits. The researchers also identified four distinct factors underlying the suits:

- The patients felt their doctors had deserted them.
- The patients felt their doctors had discounted their concerns.
- The patients felt their doctors had not provided adequate information.
- The patients felt their doctors did not understand their (or their families') perspectives.

Some of the most dramatic evidence revealing the effect of the patient-doctor relationship on malpractice claims comes from Gerald Hickson, M.D., and his research group at Vanderbilt University Medical Center. They set out to examine the association between unsolicited complaints about a physician, as recorded by Vanderbilt's patient affairs office, and that same physician's malpractice experiences. The authors concluded that a relatively small number of physicians generated a disproportionate share of complaints. They also found that a history of numerous complaints was an indicator that a physician runs a higher risk of being sued. In their words:

> *Results are consistent with previously published research on the relationship between patients' dissatisfaction with care and malpractice claims. Patients who saw physicians with the highest number of lawsuits were more likely to complain that their physicians would not listen or return telephone calls, were rude, and did not show respect.*

Risk [of being sued for malpractice] seems not to be predicted by patient characteristics, illness complexity, or even physicians' technical skills. Instead, risk appears related to patients' dissatisfaction with their physicians' ability to establish rapport, provide access, administer care and treatment consistent with expectations, and communicate effectively.

a case of failing to say *i'm sorry*

She was an extremely fit, slender, 24-year-old female who presented with classic symptoms of appendicitis: pain in the lower right abdomen, nausea, fever, and an elevated white blood count. After obtaining informed consent, I took her to the O.R. to do an exploratory laparoscopy, expecting it to result in laparoscopic appendectomy. Because I was operating in a teaching hospital, I allowed a third-year surgical resident to make the umbilical incision—not an unusual degree of responsibility for his position. His technique was not perfect and, after inserting the laparoscope, what we saw would make the heart of any surgeon skip a beat: an abdomen filling with blood from an injured artery.

We quickly converted to an open surgical procedure by making a full incision. A vascular surgeon soon arrived and controlled the accidental puncture wound with two stitches. We explored the patient's abdomen to ensure no other injuries had occurred, then performed the appendectomy and closed. Afterward, I spoke candidly with the family about what had happened, telling them this was obviously not a planned outcome or result. The patient had a rough couple of days, and I had to admit her into the intensive care unit. Her hospital stay lasted nine days.

During follow-up visits, the patient was very concerned about the scar, despite the fact that it was healing fine—from my point of view. I offered to refer her to a plastic surgeon. On the third and final follow-up visit she complained that her "insides felt all jumbled up." Since this was a non-specific complaint from a scientific standpoint, I dismissed it with the simple reassurance that it would get better with time. I said she could call me with questions any time and discharged her from my care.

The next time I heard from her, it was in the form of a malpractice suit. I was incredulous! How could she do this when I had saved her life? After much discussion with my attorney and malpractice insurer, we decided to fight the case. I was delighted that we were going to defend and deny this claim. If I'd had any idea what was to come, I would not have been so gleeful.

The legal depositions began months after the actual events. As I grew increasingly anxious about the suit, I began to see my patients in a much different light than before. I perceived each one as a possible adversary. I began habitually working out strategies for defensive recordkeeping in my head, so I would be in an advantageous position in the event of another suit. My job was no longer about care; it was about defense. It was no longer about trust and open discussion with patients; it was about cautious commentary and limiting my exposure to risk.

On the first day of the trial, my retired parents, brother, several friends, and partner attended to provide moral support. I needed it. My introduction to trial law began with 45 minutes of opening arguments in which the plaintiff's counsel derided me for incompetence as well as disregard for truth and patient welfare. He told jurors that I had committed fraud and breached my duty as a physician. He didn't merely question my character. He annihilated it. By the end of the opening arguments, my head was reeling.

The plaintiff—my patient—testified to all sorts of things regarding her care, but it was her response to the question of why she had sued that absolutely floored me: *I sued because he acted like what happened to me was no big deal. One time when I saw him in the office after this happened, he actually put his feet up on the desk while we talked. He just didn't care.*

That comment hit me like the heat from a blast furnace. It wasn't the injury and outcome that had led to that miserable day in court—it was her perception that I didn't care. My actions had communicated apathy, and that was what had landed me in court, not the medical complication.

After two weeks of intense legal debate, we won the case. But although we prevailed in battle, I still felt as if I'd lost the war. The emotional trauma of the ordeal lingered long after the case was closed. My most difficult memory surrounding the event was the reaction of my father, a physician who had practiced for over 40 years without a single malpractice claim and the man I admire more than anyone else on earth. While my attorneys were congratulating each other, he approached me and said: *I love you with all my heart, Mike, but if you ever have to go through this again, I will not be here. I will never again willingly listen to people talk about one of my children as they have talked about you these past two weeks. It is the hardest thing I have ever done, so please don't ever ask me to do this again.*

What did I learn from all this? I think the entire experience made me begin to ponder exactly how and when the entire medical profession had lost a very basic form of human kindness: the ability to offer a heart-felt, authentic *I'm sorry.*

roadblocks to apology

Many factors contribute to the problem physicians have with apology, but the most glaring is the perception that offering an apology to a patient comes with legal liability. This has created the "deny and defend" culture of medicine that I, too, was caught up in prior to my malpractice experience. The malpractice insurance industry and defense attorneys who represent physicians in malpractice cases created this culture. The lawyers are prone to warning doctors that patients and families may "misinterpret" a physician's sincere attempt to show compassion or regret.

However, there is less data to support this assumption than its alternative—that apology is actually helpful in reducing liability. In fact there may be thousands of instances each year in which a claim is not filed due to a physician's genuine expression of regret. Still, physicians continue to tell me that when they received a letter of complaint from a patient, their malpractice insurance companies or attorneys told them to stop any and all communication with the patient. I was, in fact, told this very thing by my insurer when I was sued.

Another stumbling block to apology is the medical profession's ill-conceived concept of "perfectionism." For the past 30 to 40 years, medical schools have trained physicians to believe they must make faultless decisions. People who are taught they are capable of making a perfect call every time are basically programmed to meet an unfavorable outcome with denial. They think, *It was clearly unavoidable—an act of God for which I couldn't possibly be at fault. Why should I apologize?*

In my book "The DEPO Principle," I describe seven qualities that are essential to success in medicine but that are unintentionally discouraged by medical schools and residency programs. These are summarized below.

1. DESIRABLE QUALITY
SEEKING WIN-WIN SOLUTIONS

BARRIER TO DEVELOPMENT
From start to finish, medical students compete against each other—for acceptance into the best schools, class ranking, desirable residency slots, and so on. The system is designed to winnow out the weakest at each step of the way. As a result, it teaches doctors that it's better to win than to lose, creating a culture where competition reigns supreme over cooperation.

(In contrast, MBA students are taught teamwork and interpersonal skills to prepare them for a life of leading others.)

2. DESIRABLE QUALITY
RESPECT FOR EVERY INDIVIDUAL

BARRIER TO DEVELOPMENT
Starting out at the bottom of the proverbial ladder, medical students are often belittled and sometimes even abused by the interns, residents, and attending physicians above them. As they advance, it's always clear that their rank within the hierarchy is based on being both superior and subordinate to different sets of people and that they'll be shown little respect from anyone who's attained a higher rank.

3. DESIRABLE QUALITY
PERSONAL LEADERSHIP

BARRIER TO DEVELOPMENT

Physicians develop a belief throughout their training that because they have a modicum of control over others—patients, nurses, etc.—they are "leaders." Yet true personal leadership, according to the model used in business and other industries, stresses the ability to foster teamwork and high-trust environments, not to issue marching orders.

4. DESIRABLE QUALITY
FLEXIBILITY

BARRIER TO DEVELOPMENT

As noted above, physicians advance through a well-established hierarchy during their educations. Hierarchies are by definition inflexible. They are based on doing things in a "command and control" manner.

A reliance on hard data and skepticism of softer sciences—or of anything that isn't duplicable and empirical—also leads to a rigid attitude and narrow approach that can impede problem solving.

13

5. DESIRABLE QUALITY
TEAMWORK

BARRIER TO DEVELOPMENT

As noted above, the "win-lose" model of the medical education teaches competition over cooperation. As a result, physicians tend to value autonomy. Many are uncomfortable leading, following, or even trusting their peers.

Placing a high value on winning can also lead doctors to challenge anyone who disagrees with them, creating an atmosphere of distrust.

6. DESIRABLE QUALITY
DEVELOPING OTHERS

BARRIER TO DEVELOPMENT
Working in a culture of perfectionism leads to berating rather than educating people who make mistakes. (Contrast this to business environments, where training programs are built around coaching to enhance positive behaviors.) In such a culture, feedback becomes offensive instead of instructive and constructive. It's likely to elicit defensive behavior in the recipient.

7. DESIRABLE QUALITY
OPENNESS

BARRIER TO DEVELOPMENT
Due to their training, many physicians have trouble assessing themselves accurately and receiving constructive feedback. The narrowness of their medical education also presents problems for many doctors. Medical students are taught science nearly exclusively. The liberal arts are largely excluded from their education. This tight focus results in a kind of forced social illiteracy. There's no time to learn about anything else, and the world gets a little smaller. Unfortunately, this closed-mindedness to new ideas can diminish a physician's humanity, infusing doctors with a kind of clinical detachment that hampers relationships with patients.

Author and psychotherapist Beverly Engel has noted that individuals who have difficulty apologizing possess the following traits:

- Perfectionism
- The need to be right
- Difficulty empathizing
- A tendency to be judgmental
- A willingness to project blame onto others

It's almost uncanny how Engel's list aligns with mine. No wonder the simple words "I'm sorry" are among the hardest for doctors to say. An ordinary apology of the sort delivered routinely in the course of daily life can trip up the most skilled surgeon. It can confound medical practitioners who possess some of society's most brilliant minds. In their role as healers, doctors should be master empathizers. But the same medical training that taps so effectively into their intelligence inadvertently fosters in them a kind of anti-empathy that can undermine their performance on the job.

Defining 'Professionalism'

Offering an apology following a negative outcome that might have profoundly altered the course of a patient's life should be a key component of medical professionalism. I raise this suggestion at a time when the current spotlight on "professionalism" in medicine is very intense. Not terribly focused, but certainly intense. A variety of organizations are expending energy on figuring out how best to define, characterize, categorize, and teach professionalism. It illustrates a classic tendency of the medical profession—the never-ending attempt to define everything in logical, tangible terms.

But I believe a precise definition of professionalism will ultimately elude us, because the concept embodies a collection of qualities that each defies definition and measure. Yet we all know when we observe unprofessional behavior. And since that's the case, wouldn't it be a simpler strategy to promote professionalism by targeting and addressing its antithesis, instead of trying to teach something that defies definition?

Medical schools and continuing education programs advocate ethics and professional standards on a regular basis. Still the profession as a whole demonstrates an unwillingness to identify and amend behaviors that may have become common practice, but are inherently unprofessional nonetheless.

Part of this reluctance is a failure to apologize when contrition is clearly appropriate. Nearly every other industry considers it not only fitting, but also an important part of professionalism and good customer service to express regret and offer a suitable remedy when a client is dissatisfied.

At a seminar I once attended, I heard a definition of professionalism that I've always remembered for its simplicity and universal pertinence to a wide variety of jobs. It's actually not a definition so much as a trio of behaviors that espouse personal leadership—professionalism is simply the confluence of commitment, caring, and competence. For physicians, the importance of each of these terms may not be so self-evident. Doesn't competence in medicine entail caring? Doesn't "care" refer to the processes of examination, diagnosis, and treatment planning—all of which require clinical competence and skill?

The act of caring for someone requires more than just detached, clinical attentiveness. It requires seeing the patient as a whole person with unique needs, goals, fears, and levels of health literacy. The ability of a physician to communicate caring—through empathetic words, a reassuring pat on the hand, or a compassionate look—is truly a requirement of professionalism, one that's too easily overlooked in these days of managed care, where efficiency means seeing more patients in less time and ordering fewer tests and procedures.

Apology is a key way to communicate to a patient that she matters and that you care about her. So, acting in a professional manner includes offering an apology when there has been a violation of trust, unexpected outcome, or error. Apology is just as vital to professionalism in medicine as it is in other businesses—probably more so, considering the higher stakes involved.

The business world has internalized a truth that medicine has yet to discover and embrace: Apology isn't about money or being right or wrong—for either the buyer (patient) or the vendor (doctor). It's about the provider showing respect, empathy, and a commitment to patient satisfaction; and about those receiving the apology having the grace to see the provider as human and fallible—and worthy of forgiveness.

How We Left Our Hearts to Medicine

Medicine's myopic focus on objectivity distances doctors from their patients in harmful ways. This separation is particularly damaging when a patient is in intensive care or requires heightened and detailed attention to the medico-physical aspects of care. Patients in these situations need reassurances and handholding—but unfortunately it is during such critical times that physicians believe it is especially important not to become emotionally involved with them.

Not a shred of evidence supports the concept that an individual cannot be both objective and empathetic at the same time. It isn't even logical to assume that being emotionally available to a patient will adversely affect the quality or objectivity of a doctor's clinical decision-making. But it is safe to assume that the effort to maintain an objective demeanor while discussing an unexpected outcome often registers as coldness and lack of caring. This is a dysfunctional posturing that only serves to distance the physician from the patient at a time when the latter's emotional need is greatest.

Medicine's skeptical attitude toward the softer sciences—psychology, sociology, cultural anthropology, etc.—is part and parcel of the mindset that erects barriers between physicians and the people they treat. Trained in the so-called "hard" sciences (and doesn't this terminology speak volumes?), physicians tend to be cynical about subjective approaches to understanding the world. They tend to dismiss the value these other fields of study have for enriching life.

Measurable data is the altar at which we physicians worship—and, to some extent, that's with good reason. Scientific inquiry has led to medical advancements that seemed like science-fiction fantasies just a decade ago.

But outside the isolating walls of the laboratory, the routine practice of medicine cannot rely on data alone. Newtonian-linear science will only explain the scientific-technical aspects of medicine—and perhaps incompletely in the end. Hard science is silent when it comes to the humanistic-interpersonal aspects of medicine, despite the fact that most practicing physicians will acknowledge the doctor-patient relationship is an important factor in outcome.

Albert Einstein, perhaps the greatest scientific mind of the 20th century, once wrote: *Sometimes what counts can't be counted, and what can be counted doesn't count.* But medicine tries to pare everything down to its most elemental—cells, organs and systems. In the process, we too often forget about the person whose life depends on the healthy functioning of these components.

> ## Sometimes what counts can't be counted, and what can be counted doesn't count.
> —Albert Einstein

Our goal is to heal whole people, and surely they are much greater than the sum of their parts. Philip Anderson, the 1977 Nobel Prize winner in physics (again, someone from a stringent science with a great propensity for breaking things down into their elemental components) said:

> *The ability to reduce everything to simple fundamental laws does not imply the ability to start from those laws and reconstruct the universe. In fact, the more the elementary particle physicists tell us about the nature of the fundamental laws, the less relevance they seem to have to the very real problems of the rest of science, much less society.*

In other words, as medicine understands more and more about the human body and its ailments, it seems to drift further away from humanism and the very real needs of the individuals' medicine treats. As doctors, we must stop focusing exclusively on the sterile, linear-reductionist perspective and learn how to make sound scientific judgments while remaining sensitive to patients' emotional states.

This will be difficult. But if we can do it, we'll fulfill fundamental needs of both patients and physicians, because the quality of the doctor-patient relationship not only plays a significant role in healing the patient, but also in our job satisfaction.

If physical scientists such as Einstein and Anderson can see the value of the softer side of science, surely the medical profession can. Physicians must be willing to accept that some things simply can't be summarized with a number and printed on a lab report. We can't send a requisition down to the pharmacy for a STAT order of humanism, compassion, or empathy. These must come from within—not as part of a formula for "managing" a relationship, but as an authentic, heart-felt desire to recapture what the profession has lost.

Unfortunately for everyone involved, a patient is likely to view a physician's well-intentioned emotional disengagement as coldness and even of lack of caring, just when she is in greatest need of reassurance and support. As the patient grows dissatisfied—even angry—with this, the physician may have no idea there's a storm brewing. He may feel he's demonstrating compassion and concern for his patient through dispassionate, unflustered attention to the clinical hurdles that stand in the way of wellness. Yet not surprisingly, compassion felt by the physician is invisible to the patient unless those sentiments are translated into compassionate, visible actions—a gentle touch, a caring smile, the act of really listening, and perhaps an occasional, sincere *I'm sorry*.

22

our need for apology

No matter what role you play within healthcare, at one time or another you've been a consumer of medical services. Try to remember the last time a doctor apologized to you, even for a relatively minor infraction like keeping you waiting. Can you recall a single instance?

If you're a clinician, consider these questions: When was the last time you told a patient *I'm sorry*? When did you last hear another physician apologize to a patient? To a nurse? To a hospital resident? To a medical student?

23

Your Honor or Your Life

The concept of apology as we conceive it today has not always existed. It is, in fact, a relatively new social model. In the not-too-distant past, if you harmed or offended another person, a duel was the likely method of resolution. You would defend your honor and reputation with your life—or death. That was an accepted part of the social order.

Eventually people came to understand that preserving your good name did not necessarily require pistols or sharp objects. As people sought new ways to resolve personal disputes and avenge insults, the practice of apology was born. (For more about the history of apology, see "Mea Culpa: The Sociology of Apology and Reconciliation," by Nicholas Tavuchis.)

Today, certain rules are widely understood by society-at-large regarding what an apology means and when it is appropriate. Even minor infractions of etiquette often elicit an apology from the offender. When you accidentally bump into another person, don't you say, *Excuse me*? Such an apology carries three meanings: The offender (1) shows respect for the other person, (2) shows respect for the rule that was broken, and (3) admits his understanding of the rules, and in so doing promises to abide by them in the future. Most offended people accept apologies, allowing them to preserve the relationship, re-establish trust and respect, and re-enter society with their honor intact.

But physicians have been told—and have come to believe—that it is imprudent to express contrition or regret to patients in the event of an unexpected outcome. This has resulted in a sophisticated sort of social "de-evolution" in healthcare—in essence, a permissible and sanctioned loss of civility. As a result, physicians and patients must rely on dueling to settle disputes when the patient has been "offended," whether physically, emotionally, or both. These duels are called medical malpractice lawsuits, and they are the civilized equivalent of a battle to the death.

Like the duels of yore, these courtroom combats are absolute win-lose situations. Even when physicians prevail, they are never the same psychologically. Having been through the process, I can say with conviction that it takes a toll on one's soul. I would much rather avoid the duel entirely and defend my reputation instead through the simple, honorable act of an apology. I think the day is coming when more of my colleagues will choose this route as well.

> Like the duels of yore, courtroom combats are absolute win-lose situations.

Healing the Relationship is Proactive Risk Management

As physicians, we tend to think of healing in purely corporeal terms—broken bones knitting together, sutures closing a gaping wound, antibiotics staving off an invasion of rogue microbes. But apology is also about healing. Specifically, it's about healing relationships that have been damaged by any number of means. Beverly Engel provides a compelling example in her book "The Power of Apology," which she wrote after her estranged mother apologized to her out of the blue for the childhood emotional abuse she'd inflicted on Engel. After hearing the words *I'm sorry*, Engel recalls:

> *Waves of relief washed over me. Resentment, pain, fear, and anger drained out of me. Much to my surprise, those two simple words seemed to wipe away years of pain and anger. They were the words I had been waiting to hear most of my life.*

Tremendous restorative energies are released when our transgressors simply acknowledge the roles they have played in our pain. In medicine, apology has the power to repair a violation of trust (real or perceived) that results from an unexpected outcome, complication, or medical error. It can defuse the interest of a patient or his family in pursuing financial compensation as revenge for being wronged. I believe that a heart-felt apology can be helpful in any phase of the process, even after a claim has been filed.

When a physician apologizes authentically to a patient, the apology is likely to be received as a gift. It is often reciprocated by the patient's forgiveness of the physician, the restoration of trust in the relationship, and all things being equal, a lower likelihood of a lawsuit.

Of course, the act of contrition must be authentic if it is to have its intended healing effect. An apology offered purely as a risk management tool to avoid a lawsuit is nothing more than a manipulation and may very well backfire, making a situation worse.

As it's used in healthcare today, the term "risk management" is applied to defensive activities designed to prevent or reduce financial liability stemming from a patient's injury or adverse outcome. The problem with such activities is they place physicians and hospital administrators in an adversarial role with the patients they are trained to serve. Risk management, as we know it today, has little to do with respect for the patient or maintaining a trusting relationship. Instead, it is about strategizing to avoid exposure.

But authentic apology is entirely about healing the relationship and maintaining trust. It is driven by honor and ethics, not by financial self-protection. Still, there is plenty of data to support that tangible, fiscal rewards are a natural by-product of authentic apology.

Research shows that patients are less likely to consider litigation when a physician has been honest with them and expressed regret about mistakes or poor outcomes. Patients and family members who receive heart-felt apologies can be amazingly generous in their responses, sometimes even finding the grace to console a distraught physician. On the other hand, patients and families who are denied this outlet may choose to seek a very different means of healing. Believing that "revenge" will bring them peace, they choose litigation as a means of forcing the open and honest discussion they've been denied.

'We Wept Together'

The power of an honest, open relationship between a physician and a patient is illustrated by the following true story, related to me by a friend:

> One evening, as I was about to leave the office, one of my colleagues knocked on the door asking if he could see me for a few moments. As I motioned for him to sit, I could tell this was not a social visit—he appeared to be deeply troubled. After a long period of silence, he began to speak.
>
> 'David, I am terribly torn about something and I do not know what to do. I am hoping you will help me with a decision that I can't seem to make on my own.'

He went on to relate how, a few days earlier, he had delivered an infant who died a few hours after birth. The infant was the child of a woman he'd actually delivered 25 years earlier and had cared for during his entire practice. After describing some of the details regarding the infant's death, he quickly came to the point of his struggle: 'The family sent me a funeral announcement. I don't know what to do.'

His dilemma came down to this: He was reluctant to do anything that would point to his personal failure in delivering this infant and potentially increase the liability of an already high-risk situation.

At that point, I asked him to repeat some of the details of the delivery. 'Did you actually do anything wrong?' I asked. He replied, 'I've gone through the events over and over again, and I really feel the delivery went as it should have and everything that occurred afterward was unpreventable.'

Ultimately I asked, 'What does your heart tell you to do?' he said, 'You know, I really want to go to that funeral.'

At that point I told him, 'Then by all means, go.'

A few weeks later, we crossed paths. He motioned to me to come into his consult room. We sat down together and he said, 'I just wanted to tell you what happened since I last saw you. I attended the funeral and something remarkable occurred. As the service concluded and the mourners were departing, one of the family members came up to me and asked if I would stay behind so that the grieving mother and family could have a moment alone with me. As I stood hand-in-hand within this small circle, they told me how much it meant to them that I cared enough to be there to share this moment of grief with them. Then, we wept together.'

With that, he got up out of his chair, looked at me and said, 'Thanks for letting me share that with you. I had better get back to my patients.'

This case never ended up in the courts, and I'm convinced there was no lawsuit because this physician had established a trusting relationship with the family long before the incident in question took place. When a tragic outcome occurred, he remained grounded in caring and made himself available to the patient and family. His actions helped everyone heal—including him.

As this story poignantly illustrates, avoiding a lawsuit isn't the only reason to apologize to a patient. It's an act that also heals the healer. Compare the narrative above with the following about a medical resident who failed to follow up on an abnormal test result—a chest X-ray that revealed the presence of a cancerous lesion in a patient's lung. The doctor didn't realize his mistake until he opened the man's chart a year later, during a routine annual check-up, and saw the forgotten progress note about the positive X-ray. He relates:

Realizing my oversight, I immediately reported it to the residency director. In the next agonizing weeks, I spoke with a psychiatrist on the faculty, as well as with other

residents and my advisor. I discussed the situation end-
lessly with my wife, recalling every detail and wonder-
ing how I could have 'forgotten' such a critical detail.
At the same time, I skirted the issue with the patient's
son, although I indicated that something might have
been done sooner. I felt the right thing to do was to
tell the son the truth, but I was advised that doing
so would invite a lawsuit. I felt like a moral failure.

I didn't sleep at all for three days, and then only inter-
mittently. My progress note replayed itself endlessly
in my mind. I checked in frequently with my patient
to arrange chemotherapy, pain control measures,
and, ultimately, hospice care. I last visited my patient
two days before his death, which was five months
after I uncovered my mistake. He was sleeping in a
warm room in his house. His son and I watched him
for a few minutes, then we hugged and I left. I will
never forget this patient, and I think of him when-
ever I screen and examine patients, knowing that
I don't want to miss another important diagnosis.[1]

This case illustrates to me how physicians all too often allow
fear of litigation to deprive them of the healing powers of
apology. The resident acknowledged his error to his wife, his
colleagues, and his supervisor—essentially to everyone but
the two people (the patient and his son) whose forgiveness
might have released him from his emotional agony. He also
seems to have sought comfort by becoming unusually atten-
tive to the dying patient, personally coordinating aspects of
care outside his own area and even visiting the patient and

his son at their home. Yet these attempts to assuage his own feelings of guilt by somehow making it up to the patient ultimately seem to have been less effective at allowing him to "defend his honor" than a simple apology might have been.

From a risk management standpoint, if the patient or family had discovered the non-disclosure of the error, they would have felt doubly wronged and would most likely have reacted with anger. A 1992 study by Gerald Hickson, M.D., found that of 127 families who sued healthcare providers for perinatal injuries, 24 percent were motivated to litigate because they suspected or recognized a cover-up. As we'll see later, apology is best coupled with full disclosure as soon as possible after an error or unexpected outcome. This policy is slowly gaining favor among a few organizations that refer to it as "humanitarian risk management."

Regarding the anecdote about the resident above, I find it sad that this young doctor, still in a training phase of his career, didn't receive any encouragement from his teachers and role models to be open and honest with the patient and his family. It comes down once again to how we teach professionalism—is it any wonder that apology doesn't come naturally to physicians?

Of Human Bonding

Why do the simple words "I'm sorry" have such deep, extraordinary power to mend relationships. In her book, "The Power of Apology," Beverly Engel identifies five important messages that are communicated whenever they are spoken.

1. Apologizing to a person says you respect him.
2. Apologizing shows you are able to take responsibility for your actions.
3. Apologizing demonstrates you care about the way the other person feels.
4. Apologizing reveals you feel empathy for the other person.
5. Apologizing shows your desire to resolve anger the other person feels.

Respect, responsibility, caring, empathy, and dissipating anger are pretty strong medicine when applied to a physician and patient faced with an unexpected treatment outcome. Why?

Demonstrating Respect

A study at Vanderbilt University found that the patients of physicians who received frequent complaints said they felt the physicians did not respect them. These patients understandably grew angry in the event of unexpected outcomes or errors, believing they received substandard care due to lack of respect. A physician who does not apologize or otherwise express regret for a complication exacerbates such a perception when it already exists. Humanistic risk management calls for establishing rapport with the patient as quickly as possible, but it's especially critical to demonstrate empathy and respect for a patient dealing with a less-than-desirable outcome.

Taking Responsibility

When a treatment or intervention goes badly, the patient has the right to know who will be responsible. But most patients are not as interested in "responsibility" in the sense of who is to blame as they are in who will be responsible for helping them get better. A physician can—and should—assume responsibility for coordinating care, for finding out what happened and why, and for keeping the patient and family informed. Telling the patient, *I'm sorry this has happened to you and I want to assure you I'll continue to oversee your care,* can immediately alleviate the patient's fear of being abandoned during a difficult time.

Showing Compassion

When a patient experiences a negative outcome, he wants to believe his caregiver is deeply concerned. An apology lets the patient know that his troubles aren't being shrugged off. The patient senses caring not just in the words a physician delivers, but also in the eye contact, touch, and tone of voice that accompanies the apology.

However, physicians should strive to relate to their patients and earn their trust on an ongoing basis—not just in the event of an unfortunate mistake or unforeseen problem.

The following story, related by a resident during a focus group I sponsored in Chicago on doctor-patient relationships, shows why:

> When I was in medical school, a teacher told us of this one case that happened to one of his mentors. One of his patients died, and the doctor acknowledged that he'd made a mistake. Someone approached the patient's son about suing the doctor, but the son refused. He said, 'My father loved this doctor. He felt that he could call him at home anytime, day or night, with any question. There was no such thing as a dumb question. Everyone makes mistakes, and it's not this doctor's fault that he just happened to make one bad mistake. I won't sue him for that.'

Everyone makes mistakes. I won't sue him for that.

Expressing Empathy

In a series of focus groups led by physician-researcher Dr. Thomas Gallagher in 2002, participants were allowed to observe quietly and unobtrusively while several physicians discussed their experiences with medical errors. The non-physician participants later reported feeling shocked to learn just how devastated doctors felt when their actions brought about an unintended consequence. The public seldom sees this side of doctors, because too often the urge to convey empathy to the patient is thwarted by legal concerns. Yet it is a feeling that should absolutely be tapped into, as it will facilitate healing for all parties involved.

Dissipating Anger

We don't need to delve into the research literature for proof that apology dissipates anger. We simply need to recall a time when we were angry about a real or perceived transgression but decompressed when our transgressor offered an authentic apology. This is a very basic human response.

Four Motivations for Apology

I wish it were enough to simply write about the reasons apology is important. Unfortunately, many times knowing that something is important fails to inspire us to do it. In the absence of proper motivation, common knowledge doesn't always translate into common practice. For instance, a person's motivation to work out, change his diet, or quit smoking might be very different if he suffered a major heart attack at the age of 45.

Apologizing is like that, too. Without motivation, physicians are less likely to do it. The good news is, I believe most physicians are driven by an honorable set of ethics and morals. I think they care about their patients. And I believe the motivation to apologize has always existed, but for the variety of complex and interrelated reasons outlined above, the profession has been actively discouraged from it.

Engel identified four basic motivations for apology:

1. To express regret
2. To assuage a guilty conscience
3. To salvage or repair a damaged relationship
4. To escape punishment

Let's look at each one of these as it relates to instances of unexpected outcomes in healthcare.

Expressing Regret

Expressing regret is the "purest" reason for apologizing. Apology does not imply guilt or constitute a confession. If a patient is experiencing more than typical post-operative pain for a procedure, a caring physician might tell him, *I'm sorry you're in so much pain.* Obviously, the physician is simply demonstrating empathy, not assuming culpability for the pain. Such expressions of regret and empathy build trust and forge bonds of common humanity.

Physicians are also motivated to apologize when they play a direct, causal role in an unexpected outcome. Apologies in these instances can be phrased in a way that avoids assigning blame to any one individual.

Assuaging a Guilty Conscience

When a physician is responsible for an unexpected outcome, feelings of guilt may underlie her apology. If that guilt is not accompanied by a healthy dose of regret, the effect could be less than desired. Assuaging a guilty conscience is a selfish motivation, and the doctor who apologizes solely so she can sleep at night runs the risk of coming off as a whiner who's more concerned about herself than the patient's physical and emotional problems.

Preserving a Relationship

An apology is always most effective offered up front, as soon as the offending incident occurs. An apology offered later as a means of damage control is likely to be perceived as insincere. The offended party might sense the apologizer is not really sorry for what he's done but very sorry he was caught.

Risk Management

If a physician's apology seems inconsistent with her past behavior, the patient will regard it as a manipulative ploy to avoid a malpractice suit. Doctors who cultivate open, honest relationships with their patients all along can avoid this perception.

The XY Factor

One reason apology is so hard for physicians is the XY factor. For now at least, the majority of doctors are men—and men are more likely to be raised to avoid showing signs of weakness. It's ironic, but many males seem to consider saying, *I'm sorry,* to be the equivalent of admitting defeat, of rolling over and showing their throats (or exposing their hearts). Due to their socialization, men also tend to be less skilled at communication, especially when it comes to discussing feelings—the infamous Mars-Venus conundrum.

On the other hand, perhaps because of their role in the family and society as nurturers, women tend to be better communicators. Thus, female physicians have greater success connecting with their patients. A study of 667 graduates of Jefferson Medical College concluded that women valued the psychosocial aspects of medical care more than males. A larger, national survey of 2,326 physicians revealed that the women felt, on average, that they needed 15 percent more time to provide what they considered to be high-quality care.

This indicates a greater need—and skill—on the part of female physicians to foster the doctor-patient relationship. So it should come as no surprise that yet another study found male physicians were three times more likely to be sued for malpractice than their female colleagues. As women's representation in medicine increases—and this year, for the first time, the number of women entering medical schools surpassed that of men—their influence should help change medicine's perception of the doctor-patient relationship in positive ways.

> Male physicians are three times more likely to be sued for malpractice than their female colleagues.

the four "r"s of apology

According to Engel, an authentic apology has three key elements: regret, responsibility, and remedy. In health-care, a fourth must be added—one that precedes the other three: recognition of when an apology is needed.

Though knowing when to say *I'm sorry* may seem intuitive for most people, physicians, as we have discussed, are inclined to have difficulty with it. Medicine's emphasis on deny-and-defend risk management practices coupled with the attitudes that are instilled in doctors during their training can make apologizing actually seem counterintuitive for them.

The four components of apology—recognition, regret, responsibility, and remedy—all need to be present, and preferably in that order, or else the person receiving the apology will sense that something is amiss. In fact, I believe skipping any of the components has the potential to make the situation worse—for example, expressing regret to an injured patient but failing to initiate a remedy for the harm that's been done could be infuriating.

Recognition

The key to recognizing when to offer an apology is being aware of one's own feelings as well as those of the recipient. If the doctor feels regret or remorse, or senses that her relationship with the patient is on tenuous ground, these are clear internal signals that an apology may be in order. Likewise, if the patient's (or family's) body language or manner of interaction with the doctor seems strained, this can be a clue that the patient feels there are unmet expectations with regard to outcome or communication. Sometimes what patients don't say is more important than what they do, and being able to read their visual clues is critical.

Of course, in many situations it's obvious an apology is warranted, especially when the patient is dealing with an adverse outcome. In these circumstances, the doctor must recognize that fear and uncertainty are normal reactions that can cause the patient to lash out angrily. The patient may storm in demanding answers to questions that you simply can't address without obtaining some answers of your own first. It is critical that you do not become defensive, withdrawn, or evasive. Say that you hope to address all of the questions and concerns, but first you need to know more about the situation. Ask for permission to return to the questions as soon as you've learned what you need to know in order to respond adequately.

Consider saying, *I'm sorry you're upset—I'm upset about this too. I am doing everything I can to understand how and why this happened.* If necessary, excuse yourself from the room to go clarify your thoughts, gain your composure, or look up an answer to the patient's question. But avoid letting the patient leave your office unsatisfied, even it means throwing you off schedule. That could damage the relationship—perhaps permanently—and provoke the patient to consult with an attorney before you get to the "regret" phase.

While the focus of this book is apology in the context of a medical error or complication, I encourage you not to reserve *I'm sorry* just for mishaps. Expressions of regret are considered courteous behavior in many situations. Examples of when a physician should apologize include:

- Being late for a scheduled appointment
- Receiving a patient complaint about poor service from hospital or office staff
- Interrupting a patient who is speaking—even if you must take an emergency call

In the course of daily life, keep tabs on how well you recognize situations—even minor infractions—in which an apology is appropriate. Pay attention to how you use apology outside of healthcare. Do you excuse yourself when you inadvertently offend someone? Raise your voice in frustration? Remember, professionalism is a way of life, not just something to be paraded around at work.

Regret

An expression of regret informs your patient that you recognize his pain, anxiety, or fear—and that you feel badly about it. In the event of an unexpected outcome (whether or not caused by error), a simple expression of regret might go something like this:

> *I really regret this has happened. I know it's not what either of us wanted or expected, and I'd like you to know how very sorry I am for what you're going through.*

This exchange should occur immediately after you discover the complication. It allows the relationship to begin healing. A full disclosure and a remedy can come later, after you've had time to fully assess the situation. That said, these two steps should not be put off for long, or else the patient and/or family may perceive the apology as incomplete.

Responsibility

This is the step of apology that keeps insurers, health-care administrators, risk managers, and physicians awake at night. It includes accurately disclosing everything you know about the situation in question. Bear in mind that taking responsibility does not necessarily imply acknowledging that you made a mistake. The following is an example of a statement of responsibility:

> *I am responsible for your care and will find out what happened. If possible, why it happened. I will keep you posted of what I learn and how it can be used to prevent future errors. At this point, I'm not sure if I would have done anything differently, but I intend to explore this thoroughly.*

These statements are most effective when offered in the first person singular—"I"—rather than the first person plural, or what is sometimes called "the royal we." Substitute "we" for "I" in the example above, and you'll see how it depersonalizes the message and creates the impression that the physician is trying to deflect responsibility:

> *We are responsible for your care and will find out what happened—and, if possible, why it happened. We will keep you posted of what we learn and how it can be used to prevent future errors. At this point, we're not sure if we would have done anything differently, but we intend to explore this thoroughly.*

Of course, situations occur in which the physician directly or indirectly causes the problem. I am not speaking of complications due to incompetence, which are outside the scope of this book, but rather honest mistakes resulting from communication failures, technical errors due to fatigue or limited resources, or situations beyond the doctor's control, such as idiosyncratic drug reactions or unexpected anatomical aberrations. But in these situations, the physician still initiated the treatment. Regardless of how impossible the complication was to anticipate, the physician must still assume responsibility.

A statement to offer when the physician has caused the injury or unexpected outcome might be:

> *I am responsible for your care and for this regrettable outcome. The drug reaction you experienced has been reported, but it is very uncommon. I'm looking into matters to see if your reaction could have been anticipated.*

43

At this point I can't say I would have done anything differently, but I will keep you posted of what I learn.

Remedy

An authentic apology should include an offer of restitution—a remedy that corrects the error and/or prevents it from recurring. Of course, "remedy" is a dreaded word in this context. It conjures the specter of six-figure settlements or judgments. But confronting unfortunate outcomes directly and handling them with sensitivity can defuse the outrage that fuels these outlandish awards.

Gallagher identified three major questions that patients want answered following an unexpected outcome:

- What is being done to correct the problem that I now have?
- How will this affect my health in the short and long term?
- Am I going to be responsible for the cost of this error or complication?

Each of these questions reflects the patient's need for remedy. The first two can be addressed with a statement such as:

I am personally going to do everything in my power to understand why and how this happened, and I will keep you informed about what I learn. In the meantime, I have ordered antibiotics that will help. While it is still a little too early to tell, I don't think this will result in any long-term health problems—but I'll verify that with some lab tests in a week or two. I want you to know this problem occurred because of a communication error, and I'm already looking into making changes that will prevent this kind of error from ever happening again.

But the statement doesn't address who is going to pay for the cost of the error or complication. This aspect of the issue has the potential to be sticky and very expensive, but it doesn't have to be. When a patient knows his immediate costs will be covered, his interest in seeking revenge through punitive damages diminishes. Both the hospital and physician can waive fees for services, absorb the costs of further medical treatments, and pay for inconveniences suffered by the patient and his family. Later, I'll explain how COPIC Companies, a medical malpractice insurance group, has used this approach with great success.

45

Timing and Planning

An apology should be initiated as soon as possible after discovery of the infraction, error or unanticipated outcome. Delays in communication make patients and families suspicious.

Still, physicians shouldn't be in such a hurry that they proceed without careful thought and preparation. Even when the doctor has established a good rapport and trust with the patient, a poorly delivered or ill-conceived apology could unravel the relationship, particularly in dealing with severe situations.

Engel recommends pondering six steps prior to offering an apology in order to avoid delivering one that's weak and ineffective. Five of those steps are relevant to healthcare:[2]

1. Admit to yourself what has happened to the patient.
2. Ponder the ramifications of the actions or inactions that led to or caused the problem.
3. Look at the situation from the perspective of the patient and try to understand what her feelings might be (anger, fear, anxiety, pain, etc.).
4. Forgive yourself for any causal role you had in the incident (real or perceived).
5. Plan and prepare your apology.

The physician should set the tenor of the discussion from the outset. To be effective, her body language must be in synch with her words and tone of voice. Imagine a doctor standing at a patient's hospital bedside with her arms crossed and delivering an apology while gazing intermittently out the window or glancing at the TV. Not only would the apology seem inauthentic, it might actually further infuriate the patient and family members. Apology must be approached with a demeanor of humility. The doctor should sit on the bed with the patient or on a chair placed within touching distance and maintain appropriate eye contact.

Compelled Apology: Remorse on Demand

A compelled apology is one given in response to a demand, policy, or mandate. In general, there are three groups that may call for a doctor's apology: the patient, the patient's family, or a healthcare organization administrator. (I should add that I've personally seen a nurse or two demand that a physician apologize to a patient's family.) Requests for an apology that come from a hospital, clinic, or insurance administrator are often precipitated by a complaint they've received—a complaint that has them concerned about exposure.

The most critical advice I have for a fellow physician caught in this situation is not to respond immediately.

A demand for an apology can feel like an ambush.

A demand for an apology can feel like an ambush, especially if the doctor was not previously aware of the problem. Avoid the pitfall of giving a knee-jerk, defensive response. If you need time to prepare an answer, then ask for it:

> *I see that you are angry. I would like a few minutes to reflect on my performance and how it has led to the current situation. Let me think this over so I can respond thoughtfully and accurately to your concerns and offer an appropriate apology.*

A note of caution: If you use this approach and tell patients or family members that you'll return in a few minutes, keep your promise. Don't return 20 minutes or half an hour later. They will probably be watching the clock, and your tardiness could be perceived as yet another violation of trust. It may be all that's needed to provoke them into calling an attorney.

From what I've observed, the filing of a claim often is not triggered by an isolated incident, but rather by a consistent pattern of small violations of trust and insensitivity that were tolerated until the proverbial final straw landed on the camel's back. In other words, a patient who seems suddenly to have turned on you—who is standing in your office and angrily demanding an apology—might have been dissatisfied for a while. Now he's finally venting his pent-up ire and frustration over what might seem like a relatively minor infraction. Physicians can avoid these situations by making it a habit to always treat their patients with honesty and respect, including offering apologies when they are in order rather than waiting until they are ordered.

So, what if you take the time out to ponder the situation and simply cannot figure out what the patient or family is angry about? What if you don't know what you're being asked to apologize for? Be honest:

> *I appreciate the time you gave me to reflect on things. I understand you are angry, but I am embarrassed and upset to admit that I am not sure what you are angry about. Help me understand your perspective, so I can make things right by you and ensure I don't make the same mistake again.*

In this scenario, not only does the physician recognize the patient's disappointment, but also asks for the patient's help in understanding the situation. This scenario also introduces the "remedy" step from the apology process (*...so I can make it right by you, and make sure I don't make the same mistake again...*) to further calm the angry party.

the ethical debate about disclosure

Can apology alone salvage the relationship between a doctor and a patient who's experienced an unexpected outcome? As we have seen, patients also want to know—and have a right to know—the details of what went awry when a medical intervention leaves them sicker than they were before treatment.

In medicine, reconstructing the events leading up to an adverse outcome is a process commonly called "disclosure." Unfortunately, that term has negative connotations in society-at-large, where it's used to describe the revelation of sordid—or at least unflattering—personal information. For this reason, I prefer to use the phrase "statement of transparency," which reflects honesty, openness, and a proactive willingness to share information with patients—including details that may not shine a flattering light on the healthcare provider. From this point on, when you see the phrase "statement of transparency," keep in mind that I'm referring to disclosure.

There are two major reasons why making a statement of transparency is important. First of all, it's the right thing to do ethically. Secondly, the medical profession is being mandated to inform patients about the details of adverse events.

The Patient Perspective on Disclosure

Research data show that patients want to know about bad outcomes and medical errors, even those that don't cause serious or lasting harm. Interestingly, but not surprisingly, Gallagher found that while patients identify "truthfulness" and "compassion" as having primary importance in the disclosure process, physicians say "truthfulness" and "objectivity" are the qualities that matter most. Gallagher's focus groups revealed that patients overwhelmingly want to know:

- What happened?
- How will this affect my health in the short term? In the long term?
- Why did this happen?
- What is being done to treat the problem I have now?
- Who will bear the cost of this error or complication?
- What will you do to protect other patients from a similar mistake?

Gallagher's findings are supported by research conducted by Leonard J. Marcus, Director of the Harvard School of Public Health's Program for Healthcare Negotiation and Conflict Resolution. Marcus analyzed transcripts of mediation sessions in an effort to determine what patients really want, and he discovered three main requirements: an explanation of what happened, an apology, and assurances that changes would be made to protect other patients from the same kind of harm.

Conspicuously absent from both lists is the desire to know who caused the problem.

Gallagher's focus groups revealed that patients want the doctor to take the initiative to explain situations to them. They don't want to have to interrogate the physician to get the whole story. While many physicians are wary of revealing information due to concerns about litigation, patients seek explanations not to affix blame, but simply because they want to understand. After all, their health is in jeopardy.

Note that not a single doctor in Gallagher's focus groups said he or she would offer a patient, in the aftermath of an error, an explanation about steps that would be taken to prevent similar mistakes in the future. Yet this is something patients have indicated they want to hear. And I can understand why! Not only does talking about the prevention of future slip-ups put the discussion in a more positive light, it allows people who've had these experiences to make sense of them—to take comfort in knowing that others may benefit from their distress. If there is a silver lining to the dark cloud of medical errors, it's that they can expose flawed policies and procedures, serving as a catalyst to make healthcare safer.

The Code of Medical Ethics Demands Disclosure

Ethics, compassion, caring, concern, and the avid pursuit of always doing right by patients theoretically drive the profession of medicine. Yet many physicians may not know what medical organizations have to say about honesty in communicating errors or complications to patients. The AMA has had a "Code of Medical Ethics" for some time. Section 8.12 states:

> *It is a fundamental ethical requirement that a physician should at all times deal honestly and openly with patients. Patients have a right to know their past and present medical status and to be free of any mistaken beliefs concerning their conditions. Situations occasionally occur in which a patient suffers significant medical complications that may have resulted from the physician's mistake or judgment. In these situations, the physician is ethically required to inform the patient of all the facts necessary to ensure understanding of what has occurred. Only through full disclosure is a patient able to make informed decisions regarding future medical care.*

> *Concern regarding legal liability that might result following truthful disclosure should not affect the physician's honesty with a patient.*

Please note this specific phrase: *The physician is ethically required to inform the patient of all the facts necessary to ensure understanding of what has occurred.* If a patient has an unexpected outcome, he or she has the right to know what happened, why it happened (to the extent known), and what is being done to rectify the situation. I don't believe physicians expect anything less when members of their families suffer complications.

Also note the last sentence of the AMA's code: *Concern regarding legal liability that might result following truthful disclosure should not affect the physician's honesty with a patient.* This statement presents an interesting conundrum for physicians, since many medical malpractice insurers will cancel their policies for providing full disclosure if a case ultimately lands in court. This highlights yet another situation in medicine where there is a misalignment between what people want from physicians and what they get. The good news, of course, is that evidence suggests a malpractice claim is less likely to be filed if a physician has provided a statement of transparency as part of an apology.

Disclosure is Ongoing Informed Consent

Informed consent is the process by which a fully informed patient participates in making decisions regarding his medical care. It stems from a patient's legal and ethical right to choose what happens to his body, and it should be characterized by mutual respect and shared decision-making. Informed consent is the vehicle by which patients express their personal treatment preferences and maintain their autonomy. Informed consent should include:

- A detailed explanation of the treatment, procedure, or decision in question
- Options for alternative treatments
- The benefits, risks, and uncertainties surrounding each treatment option

Ideally, before initiating treatment, the patient would be made to understand the options given, assess each one, and then select the preferred option.

As I noted earlier, lawsuits result from unmet patient expectations. The consent process is the time for physicians to have frank, clearly articulated conversations with patients regarding their expectations as well as potential risks and complications. If a patient has expectations the physician considers unrealistic, those should be clarified before proceeding.

The legal standard of informed consent has varied through the years. Its history is as follows:

The Past: The legal standard applied to informed consent in the past mandated that the information given was what a reasonable and prudent physician would tell a patient. This, obviously, gave more weight to what the physician thought was important than what the patient might want to know. This standard was not designed to empower the patient and did not respect her autonomy.

The Present: The present legal standard for informed consent states that the information provided should be what reasonable patients need to know in order to make a rational decision. This is a more patient-centered, respectful approach that strives to preserve patient autonomy. The phrase "need to know," however, still sets a physician-determined limit on what is disclosed to the patient.

The Future: The emerging standard for informed consent is the ideal—a patient-specific, subjective standard. This standard requires physicians to ask themselves *What information does this specific patient need to know and understand to make a decision?* It eliminates the concepts of "reasonable" or "average" patients and requires information to be tailored specifically to an individual. It takes into account that different patients may want to hear very different levels of detail, depending on their values, goals, cultural biases, and capability to understand clinical information. This standard obviously requires the greatest amount of skilled communication from the physician.

Obviously, when complications arise or errors occur, a patient's expectations regarding her prognosis must necessarily change. Decisions concerning care will have to be revisited—and in those instances, disclosure acts as ongoing informed consent.

Direct analogies can be made between the histories of informed consent standards and disclosure standards. Since we're talking about disclosure as an extension of the consent process, let's take a look at these:

The Past Standard of Disclosure: Prior to the litigious environment of the last 20 years, the standard for disclosure might have been described in terms similar to the past standard for consent: what a reasonable and prudent physician would tell a patient. This resulted in the patient receiving only a minimum amount of information. Compounding the problem was the typical patient's unwillingness to confront the physician or request information—that was the era when doctors were gods (well, authority figures at least). Picture a physician patting a patient on the head and saying, *Don't worry—we'll take good care of you*—and you have a good idea of just how this past standard played out.

The Present Standard of Disclosure: Too many doctors and hospitals do not even begin to fulfill the ethical consent standard of "what reasonable patients need to know to make a rational decision." Sometimes the health provider's approach is to keep information away from the patient—or to provide only the minimum required to satisfy the patient's questions. This mindset is based on a flawed view of risk management and it places the physician (or his organization) in an adversarial role with the patients in her care. It could be argued that this has been and continues to be a period of little-to-no meaningful disclosure.

The Evolving Standard of Disclosure: The emerging state of disclosure, a "statement of transparency," as mentioned earlier, is both similar to and different from the informed consent processes described above. While the amount of information and detail that individual patients wish to know about an unanticipated outcome or error may vary, one thing is clear: Everyone has the right to hear an apology, to be informed of what can be expected in the near- and long-term future, and to be reassured that he will not be abandoned.

A Lesson from the Friendly Skies

The Institute of Medicine's now infamous report on medical errors estimates that as many as 98,000 people die in hospitals each year due to medical errors. Consequently, the federal government has turned a great deal of attention to patient safety. While the IOM report recommends that the federal government require public disclosure of medical errors, organized medicine has strongly resisted.

One objection is that reporting errors in public forums might lead to sensationalization by the media and unwarranted public mistrust of the healthcare system. Proponents of mandatory error reporting believe keeping sensitive information from the public could mitigate this concern. They're in favor of doing away with the culture of blame that currently exists by instituting a non-punitive, confidential system in which errors would be disclosed to authorities that would use the data in a proactive way.

The IOM's reason for recommending mandatory disclosure makes good sense. Medical errors can nearly always be traced back to a breakdown of systems as opposed to an individual human error. Healthcare is a complex arrangement of interdependent parts that provide multiple checkpoints for catching errors. For example, a pharmacist alerts a doctor that his prescribed dose is too high for a child.

But this system also provides multiple points where breakdowns can occur—for instance, a doctor is forced to make a diagnosis without reviewing past notes because a patient's chart was misfiled. Disclosing errors instead of covering them up can pinpoint and fix weak links in the system, resulting in fewer errors down the line.

The airline industry offers a compelling model of success. Airlines cannot cover up their mistakes—plane crashes are highly visible events. Yet the industry not only survives such catastrophes, it actually bolsters public confidence by revealing the details of its investigations and the resulting efforts to prevent similar mishaps. Therefore, the traveling public believes the airlines are committed to safety and has confidence that the dangers of air travel are minimal. The statistics support this: In 1976 the risk of dying in an airplane accident was one in two million. Today—despite a huge increase in the number of flights and passengers per day— the risk is one in eight million, a fourfold increase in safety.

The Aviation Safety Reporting System (ASRS), a non-punitive error reporting system administered by NASA for the Federal Aviation Administration, has contributed greatly to safety improvements in the industry. Any airline employee who makes an error or witnesses a near miss must fill out an incident report. That person's identity is removed from the report before anyone at his airline sees it, and systems experts then analyze the reports to gain insights that are incorporated into future training programs. Thanks to this system, the number of accidents attributed to both human error and system breakdowns has plummeted.

Many physicians are skeptical that a similar system could work in medicine. They fear individuals who make medical errors would be singled out and somehow punished, despite the fact the ASRS has successfully overcome all issues of confidentiality, anonymity, and retaliatory discipline in its own system. And they argue—probably correctly—that physicians would resist being singled out for additional training designed to prevent future errors. (Pilots routinely receive training about new policies and procedures designed to enhance safety when weaknesses in the system are revealed.)

I believe a system comparable to the one employed by commercial aviation would contribute to the development of a similar culture of safety in medicine. Until such time it exists, however, the use of authentic apology and statements of transparency will help rebuild the public confidence that's shaken when errors occur.

Programs that Work: Practical Lessons in Disclosure and Apology

The telltale sign of a new concept taking hold—and perhaps becoming an emerging trend—is when several large organizations develop practices based on it. I believe this is especially true in industries with a reputation for conservatism, which includes both the healthcare and insurance industries. Let's look at a couple of organizations in these two fields that are currently implementing full disclosure policies—and with impressive results.

Veterans Affairs Medical Center

The VA Medical Center in Lexington, Kentucky, once had among the highest malpractice claims totals in the VA hospital system. In 1987, after the center lost two malpractice judgments totaling more than $1.5 million, administrators decided to adopt a more proactive policy in medical cases that had the potential to result in litigation. The core concept of the new policy was to maintain a humanistic, care-giving attitude with those who had been harmed, rather than to respond in a defensive and adversarial manner.

As the policy was implemented and ethical issues regarding disclosure arose, the risk management committee had some tough decisions to make. Ultimately committee members decided the hospital had an obligation to reveal all the details of its investigations to patients and family members affected by errors or negligence, even if they otherwise would not have known that a mishap had occurred.

Basically, this is how the system works: All workers are expected to report both errors and near misses to the hospital risk management committee. When the committee receives a report, members act quickly to determine the root cause. If a patient was harmed by the mistake, the committee generates recommendations for offering aid—such as further medical treatment, assistance in filing for disability benefits, and financial compensation. At a face-to-face meeting, representatives of the hospital apologize to the patient (or family members), emphasize the organization's regret, and explain what corrective actions will take place in response. The chief-of-staff answers medical questions and the facility's attorney offers a fair settlement.

This approach has helped to defuse anger and negate the desire for revenge, which is so often the patient's motivation for litigation. It's also reduced the VA's legal fees. Patients and/or their attorneys tend to review the clinical information volunteered in good faith by the hospital and are usually willing to negotiate a settlement on the basis of calculable financial losses rather than on the potential for large judgments that might contain punitive damages. The VA's data suggest that apology and good faith go a long way toward mitigating losses. In fact, this policy of disclosure has been so successful and has so greatly benefited the hospital financially that it has been adopted by the entire system of VA hospitals. In 1999, a retroactive study examining the seven-year period from 1990 through 1996 found there had been 88 malpractice claims against the VA medical center, but the average payment was only $15,622. In contrast, the National Practitioner Data Bank reports that nationally the mean malpractice payment for 2001 was $270,854.

The authors of the VA study acknowledged that barriers exist to adopting similar approaches at non-governmental hospitals and that private malpractice insurers, who are interested in paying as little as possible, might be inclined to resist such a strategy. However, the COPIC Companies, a medical malpractice insurance group, adopted a similar approach and achieved results that exceeded expectations.

COPIC Insurance Company

COPIC, a medical malpractice insurance company that's based in Denver, noted a basic recurring pattern in medical malpractice cases over a 30-year period. The sequence looked something like this:

1. The patient suffered a serious, unexpected outcome.
2. The patient was shocked by the failure to meet her expectations.
3. The physician adopted a deny-and-defend attitude toward his role in the outcome.

4. When the physician failed to assume accountability for the patient's concerns and needs, the patient became angry.

5. The patient called an attorney and filed a lawsuit.

This pattern led COPIC to develop what the company calls the "3Rs Program"—a plan to prevent malpractice lawsuits. The "3Rs" include:

- Recognizing that the patient has been harmed
- Responding as quickly as possible after the event
- Resolving the patient's medical issues and personal needs

COPIC-insured physicians who participate in the "3Rs Program" agree to call COPIC within 72 hours of making an error or encountering an unanticipated outcome. COPIC specialists then help the physician coordinate a face-to-face meeting with the patient to discuss what went wrong, why it went wrong, and what to expect in the near and long term. Until the medical issues have been resolved, COPIC pays the patient's out-of-pocket expenses plus $100 per day and helps arrange for things such as plane tickets for family members who need to be with their loved one.

> Of the first 80 cases COPIC ran through the program, only two resulted in further legal action.

Of the first 80 cases COPIC ran through the program, only two resulted in further legal action—a success rate that far exceeded the company's goals. I believe the main reason the program works is that it promotes honest and open communication, including what is, in essence, an apology along with a statement of transparency. It seems doubtful the program would be nearly so successful at avoiding lawsuits if money were offered without the physician's explanation and apology.

While both the VA and COPIC programs are viewed favorably because of their results and what they have taught about the power of disclosure, they are based upon, in essence, "compelled apology"—that is, apology that is mandated. The primary focus of these programs is risk management, not apology for apology's sake. I believe that spontaneous, authentic apology, offered as a genuine attempt to heal the physician-patient relationship, would be even more effective. At any rate, these two groundbreaking programs should help dispel the myth that apology and disclosure contribute to litigation.

Apology, Liability and the Law

While it is not yet a trend, legislators are beginning to remove some of the stumbling blocks to apology. At the end of the last decade, both legal academicians and policy makers began to raise the question *Should apologies be admissible into evidence as proof of fault in civil cases?*

Apology laws—laws that deny the admissibility of an apology to support a claim—have been around for some time. In the 1970s, the daughter of a Massachusetts state senator was struck and killed by a car. The father was angry that the driver never expressed any remorse, but soon learned that under then-existing evidence laws, the driver dared not apologize because it could have constituted an admission of fault. Years later the senator sponsored a bill that ultimately came to exclude "expressions of sympathy and benevolence" made after an accident to prove liability in a civil suit.

Benevolent gestures are defined as actions that convey a sense of compassion or commiseration. Examples include verbal expressions of apology or regret; written messages, including sympathy cards; and respectful conduct, such as sending flowers or attending a funeral or memorial service.

Texas passed a similar law in 1999 and California in 2000. A handful of other states followed. These laws were not specific to medical errors but to accidents in general. As written, however, slight differences in the phrasing of an apology could have a profoundly different effect on litigation. Certain kinds of apologies were protected and others were not—saying, *I'm sorry you were hurt*, for example, carried completely different legal ramifications than saying, *I'm sorry I hurt you.*

Today there is ongoing debate among legal scholars and policy makers as to whether all sorts of apologies—including those that hint at personal fault—should become inadmissible evidence in civil lawsuits. In 2003, Colorado became the first state to pass a law specific to medical apology, making statements of contrition by doctors inadmissible to support claims of physician liability. I believe other states will follow, and I hope that risk management with a humanistic approach will someday become the norm.

boot camp for authentic relationships

Patients might not be able to quickly gauge whether a physician is competent in her specialty, but they know almost immediately whether they're inclined to like her. This is important, because the nature of the doctor-patient relationship affects the quality of healthcare, and the initial interaction between a doctor and patient can set the tone for their relationship.

Sincerity—or the seeming lack of it—is one of the first quali-
ties a patient is likely to sense in a doctor. Sincerity shows in a physician's genuine, authentic attempts to see, listen to, speak to, understand, and connect with the patient. "Authentic" here means conveying a genuine interest in and respect for the individual. This is something that cannot be faked by using a communication technique learned as a risk management strategy.

Authentic communication includes the kind of informational transparency that I discussed earlier, but it is much more than that. It is bi-directional interaction between two people that begins the moment eyes meet and evolves into a complex, multi-dimensional experience. Authentic communication involves not only speech but also much subtler cues, including body language. While much of the responsibility for clear communication falls to the physician, it is a two-way street.

Seeing Authentically

To establish effective communication, physicians must understand the context of the patient's situation—not only medically, but socially and culturally as well. On first meeting patients, physicians should look for visual signs of their lifestyles: How is the patient dressed? Does he look you in the eye? What about hygiene? Is he visibly in pain or fearful? Such observations can help a physician determine a patient's health choices and health literacy—his ability to express himself and formulate questions, as well as to understand clinical explanations. Considering that one in every five patients walking into a doctor's office has poor health literacy, it only makes sense for physicians to pay attention to these clues.

This is terribly important, because the evolving standard of informed consent requires physicians to tailor the information dispensed to the individual patient's needs. And the patient's ability to understand and follow instructions will determine how faithfully he complies with the prescribed treatment plan, affecting both outcome and safety. In one study of pediatric patients, 35 percent of adverse outcomes were attributed at least partially to communication failures between clinicians or between clinician and parents.

Patients formulate their first impressions of a doctor through visual perceptions. As consumers contracting for a service, they are very likely to notice whether the provider seems respectful. A physician who neglects to maintain eye contact and stares at the patient's chart or takes notes incessantly throughout the visit comes across as closed off to the patient.

Patients want and deserve the full attention of their doctors, and they may understandably grow resentful and dissatisfied when they don't get it. They may also feel distrustful toward a physician who appears fatigued, disheveled, or distracted.

Speaking Authentically

Arguably the most important component of patient-physician communication is speech. Few things will derail the physician-patient relationship more surely than an introduction consisting of a half-hearted, limp handshake accompanied by a cheerless *Hello, I'm Dr. So-and-So* that sounds like a voice-mail recording.

I personally believe that physicians should introduce themselves by first name. I always encourage patients to call me "Mike," not "Dr. Woods." Many doctors disagree with me on this, but I know from conversations with patients that it helps put them at ease. It levels the playing field, putting doctor and patient on the same plane. Insisting on using a title constructs a barrier to open, authentic dialogue. Physician-researcher Howard Waitzkin, M.D., found that doctors often maintain a style of "high control" when communicating with patients. Elevating themselves with titles is part of this manipulation. Frankly, the days when patients held physicians in reverence and awe are gone.

Many physicians use intimidating question-and-answer techniques to maintain control—although they may not be aware that's what they're doing. Most office visits begin with an exchange of information. But often, physician-initiated questions come in machine-gun fashion and focus only on the main complaint. Few pauses are provided for the patient to respond fully. One study demonstrated that physicians on average give patients only 22 seconds to answer a question before cutting them off.

> One study demonstrated that physicians on average give patients only 22 seconds to answer a question before cutting them off.

It is not uncommon these days for physicians to rely on interview notes taken by nurses as a substitute for personally hearing the patient out. As healthcare becomes increasingly consumer-driven and the World Wide Web makes medical information ever more easily accessible, patients will have more questions than ever before. They will expect their doctors to discuss their conditions with them in detail, without having nurses or office staff act as intermediaries. Doctors should offer this without waiting for their patients to request it.

It is absolutely critical to patient care, compliance, and safety that physicians respond to patients at their level of understanding. Never dispense a prescription without first ascertaining that the patient knows what it's for. A man given medication for hypertension needs to know that hypertension means high blood pressure, which carries an increased risk of heart attack. Don't assume that he knows this just because everyone in your acquaintance does.

On the other hand, patients with above-average intelligence

or high health literacy don't appreciate being talked "down to." Waitzkin, in his study on doctor-patient communication, noted that doctors tend to underestimate the patient's desire for information. Those who have the ability to understand clinical explanations often want to hear an exact diagnosis, so offer to write down the medical terms that describe their illness and explain the diagnostic tests that will be used. Physicians who insist on using either tech talk or baby talk with patients are, frankly, attempting to maintain a controlling position. While it may take some innovative, on-the-feet thinking to adjust clinical explanations to an individual's specific level of understanding, physicians should make the effort.

Listening Authentically

Authentic listening requires listening not only with your ears, but also with your heart to comprehend the feelings beneath the words. Kevin Cashman, author of "Leadership from the Inside Out," says this about authentic listening:

> We hear the words, but do we also 'hear' the emotions, fears, underlying concerns? Authentic listening is not a technique. It is centered in compassion and in a concern for the other person that goes beyond our self-centered needs. Listening authentically is centered in the principle of psychological reciprocity: To influence others, we must first be open to their influence.

I suspect many physicians are guilty of listening selectively for only the bits of information they deem "useful" in formulating a diagnosis. Instead, they should listen with intensity, as if it were the first time they'd ever heard such a story. This holds true even if the patient has told the same story over and over again.

Authentic listening—being able to "hear" the emotions, fears and underlying concerns, as Cashman puts it—is even more important in a medical setting in which a patient experiences an unexpected outcome or complication. The predominant emotion they're feeling is fear, but physicians may miss this if it isn't expressly verbalized. In other words, the ability to listen authentically requires seeing authentically as well.

Of course, even with the best effort and intentions, the potential for misunderstanding always exists. After all, we interpret what we hear based on our worldview. Differences in cultural heritage, spiritual beliefs, education, and socioeconomic levels between physician and patient can result in varying interpretations and perceptions of the same reality. Physicians need to be sensitive to these incongruent points of view. For example, it's easy to see how a frightened patient could regard a severe allergic reaction to a new drug as a "medical error," when the doctor in fact had no way of predicting the allergy. Hearing the fear and confusion behind the patient's questions or angry accusations can go a long way toward formulating an empathetic response.

Writing Authentically

Whenever and wherever a physician writes about a patient, the notes should be clear, honest, and respectful of the individual. Furthermore, the writing should be legible and neat. Just as the physician is accountable for learning to speak with clarity and accuracy, she is also accountable for the physical act of writing clearly and accurately. Physicians who fail to write legibly either neglect to understand or refuse to acknowledge that illegible handwriting jeopardizes patient safety.

Handwriting is a learned skill, and with focus and practice everyone can write legibly. In recognition of this, Cedars-Sinai Medical Center in Los Angeles offers a handwriting class to physicians, and Indiana University Medical School has added penmanship to its curriculum. In the end, if a physician cannot write legibly, it is her responsibility to choose another method for documentation, such as dictating an entry to the patient's record, even if she has to pay for it. The reason for clear written communication is obvious from a patient safety standpoint—both in a patient record that another clinician may have to rely on at some point and on the prescription pad, since many drugs have names that look alike.

> Indiana University Medical School has added penmanship to its curriculum.

Authentic Body Language

Have you ever found yourself trying to speak to someone who was fidgeting with a pen or a paperclip? Intermittently glancing at the TV? Flipping the pages of a magazine? What kind of non-verbal messages did you receive in these scenarios? You probably felt the other person was pretending to listen but not really hearing you at all.

When you see a patient in the office or the hospital, sit down within touching distance. The patient perceives a standing physician very differently than a physician who is seated. One study asked hospitalized patients to estimate the amount of time their doctors spent with them. All the doctors' visits lasted exactly five minutes, yet patients who saw a standing physician estimated the visit lasted about two or three minutes, while those whose physicians pulled a chair up to the bedside perceived the visit to have lasted 15 minutes. The message of the standing physician is *I'm in a hurry, so let's get this over with*! The message of the physician who sits is *I've got as much time as you need*. While in reality the amount of time spent is the same, the patient's assessment is very different.

Another critical issue of body language is eye contact. Look at your patient. Don't flip through the chart. If you typically make notes in the chart during an appointment, ask the patient if it's okay—yes, ask for permission—or do it after you leave the room. Using periods of eye contact, with appropriate pauses in between, is common social etiquette. Failure to make adequate eye contact engenders mistrust. And whether standing or sitting, don't cross your arms. It sends the message that you are trying to keep a barrier between yourself and the patient, or that you are in a hurry.

Trust Accrual and Trust Equity

Establishing a relationship with another person—any person—requires that you demonstrate trustworthiness. Once upon a time, merely having an "M.D." behind your name earned trust. Today, from a patient's perspective, the credentials behind the name do not necessarily mean anything but clinical competence—and sometimes even that is no longer assumed.

Trust is established over time. It can be challenging to gain a patient's trust in the all-too-common 10-minute office visit or hospital consult. And trust is difficult to foster when a physician does not consistently see the same patient, when there is no provider-patient continuity. In some practices it's the norm for whoever is "on" that day to see the patient in the office or hospital. Many OB/GYN groups rotate their pregnant patients through multiple partners because they rotate call. From both a relationship and risk management standpoint, this is an uncertain practice. In the event of a bad outcome, there's an increased likelihood of a malpractice claim, for the simple reason that the patient did not build a trusting relationship with the doctor she feels is responsible.

In today's healthcare environment, distrust is the norm until a patient has spent sufficient time with a doctor to establish a relationship. One approach to understanding trust is to think about it in banking terms. Trust accrual occurs over a period of time, just as a relationship is built one office visit at a time. An extended first visit is particularly helpful. The additional time spent getting to know the patient lays a foundation for trust, but remember that it's insufficient on its own. Spending time in subsequent visits and making a commitment to patient continuity will ultimately lead to trust equity.

A high level of trust that's established through repeated encounters is not likely to be wiped out with a single negative experience. The patient will be more likely to give the physician the benefit of the doubt when there is substantial trust equity to draw on. The bad experience may lower the equity in the physician's "account." But open communication and continuity with the patient will allow trust to accrue again over time—and a sincere apology will contribute to it.

It is when a patient feels abandoned and cut off from communicating with his doctor that all trust equity is likely to dissipate and the account will be closed. With nothing left to draw on, the patient may become resentful and angry, choosing other ways to settle his grievances.

Calculating Trust Equity: Tools for Physicians

Physicians can gauge how well trust equity is accruing in their patient relationships by asking themselves a few questions:

For Primary Care Givers: Can you put a face with the name of most of your patients without having to refer to the chart for identifying details? If you ran into them on the street, would you be able to greet them by name? When you can't recall a patient's name, can you at least recall something specific or unique about her? If you answered "no" to most of these questions, you might have a problem seeing and hearing authentically. You might question if you take enough time with your patients, or if you simply have too many patients. Or is lack of continuity of care, which prevents you from seeing the same patient in subsequent encounters, to blame?

For Physicians in a Referral Practice (surgeons, gastro-enterologists, cardiologists, etc.): Specialists tend to see a greater number of new patients in any given time period. This doesn't relieve them of the responsibility of establishing and maintaining trust. Continuity, on the other hand, may not be as important for you as it is for primary care givers. Physicians in referral practice should consider this question: In two years, will this patient remember my name? In other words, are you establishing an effective relationship that will cause a patient to remember you beyond the procedure you performed or the treatment rendered? The answer reflects the degree of connection that you make with your patients. I've seen patients with multiple abdominal scars from various surgeries that could not recall the names of the surgeons. How strange that someone would not remember the name of a person who operated on her? What does this say about the relationship?

Recognizing Difficult Physician-Patient Communication

Researcher Maysel Kemp White identified that there are three clues that clearly signal a difficult relationship:

- **Interruption:** either the doctor or the patient is frequently and/or increasingly interrupting the other.

- **Repetition:** either party frequently repeats the same statements, often getting louder with each repetition.
- **Stereotypical Responses:** either party (but usually the physician) responds in clichés to disengage the other party (e.g., *Don't worry about that*, or, *That's just our policy*).

'Human-Issue-Human' Approach

The "human-issue-human" approach is a useful technique for overcoming problem communications. In a nutshell, you first acknowledge the human, then deal with the issue, and close by focusing on the human again.

For example, when a patient is upset or angry, engage her as a person first and foremost. Call her by her first name if you can. Empathize with her concerns, whether voiced or observed, but reflect her feelings: *Michelle, I can see that you are very upset.* Verbal validation of the feeling gives the patient an opening to talk to you about her problem. When you demonstrate an understanding of a patient's distress, it helps her feel calmer. Once she is authentically engaged, address the problem: *Michelle, how can I be of assistance in this situation? What do you need from me now?*

If you are unable to address the issue directly, tell her you will find an answer or engage someone who will be able to help. Taking notes, as long as you pay attention and maintain appropriate eye contact, conveys that you are truly interested and intend to follow-up. Tell the patient you will contact her with your findings.

Finally, re-focus on the personal relationship. Close the inter-action: *Michelle, I'm glad you brought this to my attention. I'll do my best. Please don't hesitate to give me additional feedback.*

Conclusive Changes

Of course, I have presented here just a few of the myriad relationship-building tools that should be standard-issue with a medical diploma. As healthcare continues on its inexorable path toward becoming a more patient-centered system, the ability to establish and maintain strong, productive relationships with staff and patients alike will be essential to doctors' professional survival.

In 1998, the Accreditation Council for Graduate Medical Education adopted "interpersonal/communication" and "professional" skills as core competencies in which gradu-ates must demonstrate proficiency. As medical schools align their curricula with these competencies, young doctors will be emerging from school equipped to handle the "soft" side of medicine in a way that I believe will produce better health-care, increased job satisfaction, and lower malpractice costs.

Apology is a fundamental part of the standard reper-toire of social communication. I hope someday saying, *I'm sorry,* will be as easy for doctors as it is for the rest of the world, because it will signal that we have fully integrated our humanity into our profession.

78

appendix a

A Summary of the Authentic Apology Process

Compared with the volume of information healthcare providers are required to learn and assimilate during their education and training, there is relatively little they need to learn,
in terms of volume, regarding apology. An authentic apology
is one that is heart-felt and driven by true regret or remorse.

Author and sociologist Beverly Engel notes that there are
five reasons to apologize: Authentic apology shows the other
person you 1) respect them, 2) are taking responsibility for
the situation, 3) care about the way the individual feels, and
4) are empathetic. The fifth reason to apologize is that it dissipates anger, and disarms the individual.

The long histories of "deny and defend" risk management
practices and attitudes physicians acquire during training
(such as perfectionism and skepticism of the softer aspects
of relationships) contribute to a reluctance or inability
to recognize when an apology is needed. The ideology
of "objectivity at all costs" has hardened hearts in some
physicians, and they fail to appreciate that the patient's
emotional needs are not amenable to technology or logic.

Specific Information Patients Want to Hear

Dr. Thomas Gallagher and his colleagues, in a study of the attitudes of patients and physicians toward medical errors, found that patients want to know very specific things after experiencing a medical error or unexpected outcome:

- What happened?
- How will this affect my health in the short and long term?
- Why did this happen?
- What is being done to correct the problem that I now have?
- Am I going to be responsible for the cost of this error or complication?
- What has been learned and what are you doing to avoid having this happen again?

Beyond this, patients want—and increasingly expect—an apology.

The Five Steps of Planning an Apology

A poorly planned apology can be as bad as or worse than none at all. While Engel notes there are six steps to effective apology, only five are relevant to healthcare:

1. Admit to yourself what has happened to the patient.
2. Ponder the ramifications of your actions/ inactions leading to or causing the problem.
3. Look at the situation from the patient's point

of view and try to understand what his feelings might be (anger, fear, anxiety, pain, etc.).

4. Forgive yourself for any causal role you had in the incident.

5. Plan and prepare your apology—if necessary, write out what you intend to say, based upon the Four "R"s.

The Four "R"s of Authentic Apology

Authentic apology has four elements that are applicable to healthcare: recognition, regret, responsibility, and remedy. Briefly, each element has the following salient features:

Recognition

A doctor needs to be able to read his own feelings as well as the feelings of the patient and family. Feeling regret or remorse is a good indicator that an apology is in order. If the patient is interacting with you differently or is reluctant to talk, it may be a clue there are unmet expectations.

Regret

An expression of regret is an empathetic response that lets the patient know you understand what she's going through and that you feel badly about it. An example of a statement of regret for an unexpected outcome is: *I am so sorry. I know this outcome is not what you expected. It is not what I expected either.*

This exchange can take place immediately following the incident. It allows the healing of the relationship to begin.

Responsibility

Assuming responsibility incorporates the concept of disclosure, or what I call a "statement of transparency." A statement of transparency should include all of the specific elements patients want to know about their unexpected outcome or error: what happened, why it happened, how it will affect long- and short-term health status, and what steps are being taken to ensure it will not happen to others in the future. It is the responsibility of the physician to provide this information.

Remedy

Authentic apology requires offering a remedy, but that does not necessarily mean money. A significant part of any remedy is simply responding to the patient's following questions:

- What is being done to correct the problem that I now have?
- How will this affect my health? Short term? Long term?
- Am I going to be responsible for the cost of this error or complication?

bibliography

American College of Physicians–American Society of Internal Medicine. "Do You Need to Talk to Patients About Mistakes?" *ACP-ASIM Observer.* March 2002.

Beckman, H.B. "The Doctor-Patient Relationship and Malpractice. Lessons from Plaintiff Depositions." *Archives of Internal Medicine.* 154(12): 1365-1370, June 27, 1994.

Blanchard, Ken and McBride, Margret. *The One Minute Apology.* New York, New York: Harpers Collins Publishers Inc., 2003.

Carroll, John. "The Good Doctor." *American Way Magazine.* July 15, 2003. <http://www.americanwaymag.com/lifestyle/feature.asp?archive_date=7/15/2003> (Last accessed on April 15, 2004).

Cegala, Donald, et al. "The Effects of Patients Communication Skills Training on Compliance." *Archives of Family Medicine.* 9(1): 57-64, January 2000.

Cohen, Jonathan. "Apology and Organizations: Exploring an Example from Medical Practice." *Fordham Urban Law Journal.* 27(5): 1447-82, June 2000.

Cohen, Jonathan. "Legislating Apology: The Pros and Cons." *University of Cincinnati Law Review.* 70(3): 819-872, Spring 2002.

Cohen, Jonathan. "Advising Clients to Apologize." *Southern California Law Review.* 72(4): 1009-1070, May 1999.

Edwards, Kelly. "Informed Consent." *University of Washington School of Medicine. Ethics in Medicine.* February 22, 1999. <http://eduserv.hscer.washington.edu/bioethics/topics/consent.html> (Last accessed on December 17, 2003).

Engel, Beverly. *The Power of Apology.* New York, New York: John Wiley & Sons, Inc., 2001.

Fish, Jeremy. "Honesty is the Best Policy When Discussing Medical Errors." *AMedNews.com Ethics Forum.* November 4, 2002. <http://www.ama-assn.org/amednews/2002/11/04/prca1104.htm> (Last accessed on October 21, 2003).

Foubister, Vida. "Broadening the Role of Forgiveness in Medicine." *American Medical News.* 169, August 21, 2000.

Gallagher, Thomas, et al. "Patients' and Physicians' Attitudes Regarding the Disclosure of Medical Errors." *JAMA.* 289(8): 1001-1007, February 26, 2003.

Helmreich, Robert. "On Error Management: Lessons from Aviation." *British Medical Journal.* March 18, 2000.

Hickson, G.B., et al. "Patient Complaints and Malpractice Risk." *JAMA*. 287(22): 2951-2957, June 12, 2002.

Kaledin, Elizabeth. "What Pilots Can Teach Doctors." *CBS News.com*. December 17, 2000. <http://www.cbsnews.com/stories/2002/01/31/health/main326420.html> (Last accessed on April 15, 2004).

Kapp, M. B. "Legal Anxieties and Medical Mistakes." *Journal of Internal Medicine*. 12(12): 787-788, 1997.

Kelly-Wilson, Lisa, and Parsons, Jennifer. "Physicians and Medical Malpractice Litigation: Final Analytical Report." *Survey Research Laboratory Study #894*. 29-31, February 2003.

Kraman, Steve and Hamm, Ginny. "Risk Management: Extreme Honesty May Be the Best Policy." *Annals of Internal Medicine* 131(12): 963-967, December 21, 1999.

Levinson, W, et al. "Physician-Patient Communication. The Relationship with Malpractice Claims Among Primary Care Physicians and Surgeons." *JAMA* 277(7): 553-559, February 1997.

Lukaszewski, James. "Telling the Truth Reduces Liability? Who Woulda Thought?" *PBI Media LLC's PR News*. 2000.

Marcus, Leonard and Dorn, Barry. "Can't We All Just Get Along? Let's Talk More and Litigate Less." *AMedNews.com Professional Issues*. September 15, 2003. <http://www.ama-assn.org/amednews/2003/09/15/prcb0915.htm> (Last accessed on October 21, 2003).

Neary, Walter. "Doctors Should Consider Providing More Information to Patients About Medical Errors." *University of Washington News and Events.* February 25, 2003. <http://www.washington.edu/newsroom/news/2003archive/02-03archive/k022503a.html> (Last accessed on March 18, 2004).

Okie, Susan. "An Act of Empathy." *Washington Post.* October 21, 2003. <http://www.washingtonpost.com/ac2/wp-dyn/A55573-2003Oct20> (Last accessed on October 21, 2003).

Paulos, John. "Preventing Medical Mistakes: The Issue Goes Beyond Medicine." *ABCNews.com.* January 1, 2003. <http://abcnews.go.com/sections/scitech/WhosCounting/whoscounting000101.html> (Last accessed on December 12, 2003).

Prager, Linda. "New Laws Let Doctors Say 'I'm Sorry' for Medical Mistakes." *American Medical News.* 169, August 21, 2000. <http://www.ama-assn.org/amednews/2000/08/21/prsa0821.htm> (Last accessed on October 21, 2003).

Princeton Insurance. "Satisfied Patients Less Likely to Sue: Customer Service More Important Than Ever." *Risk Review Online.* 2002-2003. <http://www.riskreviewonline.com/1103/risk_mgt/riskmanagement_full.html> (Last accessed on April 15, 2004).

Ranum, Darrell. "Medical Error–Delivering Bad News." *RISKResource* 7(4), Winter 2001.

Robeznieks, Andis. "The Power of an Apology: Patients Appreciate Open Communication." *AMedNews.com Professional Issues.* July 28, 2003. <http://www.ama-assn.org/amednews/2003/07/28/prsa0728.htm> (Last accessed on October 21, 2003)

Shapiro, Dan. "Beyond the Blame: A No-Fault Approach to Malpractice." *The New York Times.* September 23, 2003. <http://query.nytimes.com/gst/abstract.html?res=FB081 FF7355E0C708EDDA00894DB404482> (Last accessed on September 23, 2003).

Waitzkin, H. "Doctor-Patient Communication. Clinical Implications of Social Scientific Research." *JAMA.* 252(17): 2441, November 2, 1984.

Waitzkin, H and Elderkin-Thompson, V. "Difference in Clinical Communication by Gender." *Journal of General Internal Medicine.* 14(2): 112, February 1999.

Walton, Merrilyn. "Open Disclosure to Patients or Families After an Adverse Event." *University of Sydney Faculty of Medicine Literature Review.* November 25, 2001.

Witman, AB, et al. "How Do Patients Want Physicians to Handle Mistakes? A Survey of Internal Medicine Patients in an Academic Setting." *Archives of Internal Medicine.* 156(22): 2565-2569, December 9-23, 1996.

Woods, Michael and Haygood, Martin. "The Physician Risk Assessment Development Report." Management Psychology Group. 2003.

Woods, Michael. *Applying Personal Leadership Principles to Health Care: The DEPO Principle.* Tampa, Florida: American College of Physician Executives, 2001.

footnotes

1 Albert W. Wu. "A Major Medical Error: Medical Resident Tells How He Coped With It." Reproduced with permission from the March 1, 2001, issue of *American Family Physician*. Copyright ©2001 American Academy of Family Physicians. All Rights Reserved.

2 Engel's sixth point is to "forgive the other person for harm done to you in the past," advice that's not relevant in the setting addressed here.

To order additional copies or for more information, contact:

Doctors in Touch
1100 Lake Street, Suite 230
Oak Park, IL 60301
708.697.6447
info@doctorsintouch.com

www.doctorsintouch.com

Printed in the United States
25448LVS00005B/274